Contents

0

Introduction: Embarking on Your Path to Natural Healing

Welcome to Mission to Remission, A Journey of Healing Auto Immune Conditions through Nutrition. This book provides a step-by-step guide to stopping your autoimmune condition in its tracks and reclaiming your life. It will be your companion on a transformative path towards understanding and harnessing the power of the Autoimmune Protocol (AIP) to heal, reduce pain, and regain control of your life.

If you've been struggling with an autoimmune disease, you're not alone. These conditions, such as rheumatoid arthritis, celiac disease, multiple sclerosis, and lupus, to name a few, can cause chronic inflammation, pain, and a range of debilitating symptoms. But there is hope. The Autoimmune Protocol, or AIP, is a science-backed approach that can help reduce inflammation, promote healing, and improve your overall well-being.

If you are reading this book, you have already taken the first step toward reclaiming your health. As someone who has personally experienced the challenges of living with Rheumatoid Arthritis, I understand all too well the pain you may be enduring. However, I have also come to realise the significant impact that diet has on exacerbating or alleviating that pain. And let me assure you, once you discover this for yourself, you won't need any external motivation to give up inflammatory foods. The relief from pain will serve as all the motivation you need.

Regardless of where you currently stand on your health journey, whether you have recently been diagnosed or have been struggling for a long time, now is the perfect time to initiate the healing process. This guide is specifically designed to provide you with straightforward and practical information to navigate the Autoimmune Protocol (AIP), which is widely recognized as the most effective diet for individuals with autoimmune conditions who aspire to achieve remission. This book will guide you step by step through the Autoimmune Protocol, providing practical tips, meal plans, and delicious recipes that are easy to follow. You don't need to be a gourmet chef or have a degree in nutrition to succeed on this journey.

Throughout this journey, we will explore how certain foods can trigger inflammation and worsen your autoimmune symptoms. By eliminating potential triggers, such as gluten, dairy, and processed sugars, and focusing on nutrient-dense, healing foods, you can support your body's natural healing processes.

But the Autoimmune Healing Journey doesn't stop at dietary changes. We will also explore the importance of lifestyle modifications, stress management techniques, sleep optimisation, and personalised self-care practices. These factors can greatly impact your overall health and well-being, helping you on your path to recovery.

Remember, healing takes time and dedication. But by embracing the principles of the Autoimmune Protocol, you can take charge of your health and reclaim your life.

So, let's begin this transformative Autoimmune Healing Journey together. Get ready to discover a new way of nourishing your body, supporting healing, and experiencing the benefits of natural recovery.

Chapter 1: Introduction to the Auto Immune Protocol (AIP)

The Autoimmune Protocol (AIP) is a dietary and lifestyle approach promoted by a team of medical professionals, including Dr. Sarah Ballantyne, Dr. Terry Wahls, Mickey Trescott, and Angie Alt. Dr. Sarah Ballantyne, also known as The Paleo Mom, is a well-known expert in the field of autoimmune diseases and nutrition. She is a scientist, researcher, and author who has extensively studied the impact of diet and lifestyle on autoimmune conditions.

The AIP is rooted in scientific research, case studies, and practical knowledge gained from lived experiences. It offers a comprehensive approach for managing autoimmune diseases through specific dietary and lifestyle modifications. The protocol aims to reduce symptoms and promote healing by addressing the underlying factors that contribute to autoimmune conditions. The AIP has gained significant popularity and recognition within the autoimmune community. Many individuals with autoimmune diseases have reported positive outcomes with many people achieving full remission after adopting the AIP.

The Autoimmune Protocol (AIP) is a comprehensive approach to managing autoimmune conditions by focusing on three key pillars: Sleep, Stress management, and Diet. Autoimmune diseases occur when the body's immune system mistakenly attacks its own tissues and the fail-safes that typically regulate the immune system malfunction. Factors such as inflammatory foods, stress, and lack of sleep can further stimulate the immune system, exacerbating the autoimmune response. The AIP aims to address these factors and provide a framework for healing and regulating the immune system.

One fundamental aspect of the AIP is recognizing the importance of gut health in autoimmune conditions. The lining of the gut houses approximately 70- 80% of our immune system. Its role is to absorb nutrients while preventing the entry of toxins and harmful bacterial byproducts into the body. When the gut barrier is compromised, toxins can enter the bloodstream, triggering an immune response. The bacteria residing in our gut play a crucial role in this process, aiding in digestion, nutrient absorption, and the regulation of the immune system.

The gut bacteria produce neurotransmitters, which can influence mood and behavior, as well as impact hormone production. Therefore, an imbalance in gut bacteria can have far-reaching effects on various systems in the body. The AIP diet is specifically designed not only to eliminate inflammatory foods but also to promote gut healing through the consumption of nutrient-dense foods.

The principles of the Paleo diet focus on consuming whole, unprocessed foods similar to those eaten by our ancestors. However, the AIP takes it a step further by eliminating foods that, although nutrient-dense, may still have inflammatory properties. These foods, which would typically be allowed on a Paleo diet, are removed from the AIP to support the healing process.

One crucial aspect of the AIP is addressing nutrient deficiencies that are often associated with autoimmune diseases. Vitamins such as B, A, C, E, zinc, and amino acids like glycine are essential for the proper functioning of the immune system. A nutrient-dense diet provides the necessary building blocks for the body to heal tissues and allow all systems to function effectively. Incorporating foods such as organic meat, seafood, and a wide variety of vegetables into the AIP can help achieve this goal.

In addition to dietary modifications, the AIP emphasizes the importance of adequate sleep and stress reduction. Sleep deprivation and chronic stress can negatively impact the immune system and increase the production of stress hormones like cortisol. This can further burden the immune system and contribute to autoimmune flare-ups. By prioritizing sufficient sleep and implementing stress management techniques, individuals following the AIP can support hormonal regulation and allow the immune system to function optimally.

The underlying principle of the AIP is to create an environment that promotes hormone regulation, gut health, and nutrient density. By addressing these factors, the immune system can better regulate itself and promote healing of damaged tissues. The AIP offers a holistic approach to managing autoimmune conditions, empowering individuals to take an active role in their health and well-being.

Chapter 2: Starting with Paleo

The Paleo diet serves as an excellent starting point for individuals looking to manage inflammation and promote overall health. Some people experience significant improvements in their health and even achieve full remission by following the Paleo diet alone. However, it's important to recognize that each person is unique, and their bodies may respond differently to dietary changes. To begin with the least restrictive approach, I recommend trying the Paleo diet first. Additionally, some individuals may find that they can tolerate raw dairy products.

So, what exactly is the Paleo diet? Also known as the "caveman" or "ancestral" diet, the Paleo diet focuses on consuming foods that our ancestors would have eaten during the Paleolithic era. The primary emphasis is on whole, unprocessed foods while excluding grains, legumes, dairy, refined sugars, and processed foods. By avoiding these potentially inflammatory foods, individuals aim to reduce inflammation and promote healing within the body.

Regarding dairy, the traditional Paleo diet excludes it entirely. Dairy products may contain proteins, such as casein and whey, which can trigger inflammatory responses in some individuals. Symptoms like bloating, digestive issues, skin problems, and joint pain can arise as a result.

While certain individuals may tolerate dairy without experiencing adverse effects, others may find that it exacerbates inflammation and hampers the healing process. This is especially true for individuals with lactose intolerance or sensitivities to dairy proteins. It's crucial to pay close attention to your body's signals and assess how dairy consumption impacts your overall well-being and inflammation levels.

Within the context of the Paleo approach, there is a variation that allows for the inclusion of grass-fed dairy. Grass-fed dairy products come from animals raised on a natural diet of grass and pasture, offering additional nutritional benefits. They are rich in essential nutrients like vitamins A and K2, omega-3 fatty acids, and conjugated linoleic acid (CLA). However, it's important to note that even grass-fed dairy can still contain potentially inflammatory proteins found in conventional dairy.

Understanding your body's response to dairy is a key aspect of managing inflammation and promoting healing. By closely monitoring your symptoms and overall well-being, you can determine whether dairy consumption contributes to inflammation or hinders your progress. Each person's response to dairy is highly individual, and what works for one person may not work for another.

If you suspect that dairy is causing or exacerbating inflammation in your body, it is advisable to transition to a dairy-free diet. This entails eliminating all forms of dairy, including milk, cheese, yogurt, butter, and ghee. It's important to carefully read ingredient labels, as dairy can be found in various processed foods under different names.

By following a dairy-free Paleo approach, you can further reduce potential sources of inflammation and support your body's healing process. In the subsequent chapters, we will explore the Autoimmune Protocol (AIP), a more comprehensive dietary approach specifically designed to address inflammation and promote healing.

Foods to include on the Paleo diet:

Meat: Grass-fed beef, poultry, pork, lamb, and game meats.

Fish and Seafood: Wild-caught fish, such as salmon, mackerel, tuna, and sardines. Shellfish like shrimp, crab, and lobster.

Eggs: Pasture-raised or organic eggs.

Vegetables: A wide variety of vegetables, both cooked and raw.

Fruits: Fresh fruits in moderation, focusing on lower-sugar options like berries.

Nuts and Seeds: Almonds, walnuts, macadamia nuts, hazelnuts, sunflower seeds, chia seeds, flaxseeds, etc.

Healthy Fats: Avocado, olive oil, coconut oil.

Herbs and Spices: Use a variety of herbs and spices to add flavor to your meals.

Non-Dairy Milk Alternatives: Unsweetened almond milk, coconut milk, or other plant-based milk options.

Fermented Foods: Sauerkraut, kimchi, pickles (without added sugar), and coconut milk yogurt (dairy-free).

Foods to avoid on the Paleo diet:

Dairy Products: Milk, cheese, yogurt, butter, ghee, and any other products made from cow's, sheep's, or goat's milk.

Grains: Wheat, barley, oats, rice, corn, and all gluten-containing grains.

Legumes: Beans, lentils, chickpeas, peanuts, and soy products.

Refined Sugars and Sweeteners: White sugar, brown sugar, agave nectar, and artificial sweeteners.

Processed Foods: Packaged snacks, fast food, and any foods with additives, preservatives, or artificial ingredients.

Vegetable Oils: Soybean oil, corn oil, canola oil, and other highly processed oils.

Alcohol: Beer, wine, spirits, and other alcoholic beverages.

If you choose to include grass-fed dairy in your Paleo approach, there are a few options to consider:

Grass-fed Butter: Use real grass-fed butter in moderation.

Ghee: Clarified butter with the milk solids removed, often tolerated by those with dairy sensitivities.

Grass-fed Yogurt: If tolerated, opt for plain, unsweetened yogurt made from grass-fed milk.

Certain Cheeses: Some individuals may tolerate certain types of cheese made from grass-fed milk. Examples include hard, aged cheeses like cheddar or parmesan. However, it's important to assess your individual tolerance.

Remember, if you decide to include grass-fed dairy in your Paleo approach, closely observe your body's response. If it triggers inflammation or other adverse effects, it may be necessary to eliminate it from your diet. Personalization and listening to your body's needs are key to achieving optimal results in managing inflammation through diet.

In the subsequent chapters, we will delve into the Autoimmune Protocol (AIP), which is a more comprehensive dietary approach specifically designed to address inflammation and promote healing.

Chapter 3: The Autoimmune Protocol (AIP)

Now, let's dive deeper into the AIP and provide you with a comprehensive, step-by-step approach to following the AIP diet. This chapter aims to equip you with the knowledge and tools necessary to embark on your healing journey and make the AIP a sustainable and effective part of your lifestyle.

What is AIP:

The Autoimmune Protocol (AIP) is a therapeutic dietary approach designed to reduce inflammation, support gut health, and manage autoimmune diseases. The AIP builds upon the principles of the Paleo diet and eliminates additional potentially inflammatory foods to create a stricter framework for healing. The key Principles of the AIP are to address gut health, eliminate trigger foods and introduce nutrient-dense foods.

How the AIP Differs from the Paleo Diet:

While the AIP shares similarities with the Paleo diet, it is a more restrictive and targeted approach specifically designed for individuals with autoimmune conditions. Here are some key differences between the AIP and the Paleo diet:

Elimination of additional inflammatory foods: The AIP eliminates additional foods beyond what the Paleo diet excludes. These include nightshade vegetables, eggs, nuts and seeds, coffee, alcohol, and certain food additives. These foods are known to have the potential to trigger inflammation and immune reactions in susceptible individuals.

Focus on gut health: The AIP places a significant emphasis on gut health and recognizes the role of the gut microbiome in autoimmune conditions. It encourages the consumption of gut-supportive foods, such as bone broth and fermented vegetables, to promote a healthy gut environment and reduce intestinal permeability.

Phased approach and reintroduction: The AIP often involves a phased approach, starting with an elimination phase where all potentially problematic foods are removed. After a period of strict elimination, some individuals choose to reintroduce eliminated foods systematically to identify specific triggers or sensitivities. This reintroduction phase allows for personalization of the diet based on individual tolerances and preferences.

Individualized approach: The AIP recognizes that each person's response to specific foods may vary. It encourages individuals to listen to their bodies, work with healthcare professionals or registered dietitians, and customize the protocol to suit their specific needs and health goals.

By incorporating these additional elements and focusing on the management of autoimmune conditions, the AIP provides a more targeted and tailored approach compared to the broader scope of the Paleo diet.

During the AIP journey, you may experience cravings or emotional triggers related to food. Here are some strategies to help you manage them effectively.

Coping with food cravings during the AIP journey:

Identify the root cause: Understand whether your cravings are driven by physical hunger, emotional triggers, or nutrient deficiencies. Addressing the underlying cause can help manage cravings more effectively.

Increase your protein: Protein will help promote feelings of fullness and satisfaction.

Find AIP-friendly alternatives: Explore AIP-friendly recipes or substitutes for your favorite foods. There are numerous creative recipes and ingredient swaps available that can satisfy cravings within the confines of the AIP.

Focus on nutrient-dense foods: Ensure you're consuming a variety of nutrient-dense foods to minimize nutrient deficiencies that can contribute to cravings.

Practice mindful eating: Slow down, savor your meals, and pay attention to the flavors, textures, and satisfaction derived from the foods you eat. Mindful eating can help reduce cravings and promote a healthy relationship with food.

Strategies for dealing with emotional eating triggers:

Identify emotional triggersand find alternative coping mechanisms: Recognize the emotions or situations that trigger emotional eating. Find healthier ways to cope with stress, boredom, or other emotional states. Engage in activities such as exercise, meditation, journaling, or talking to a supportive friend or therapist.

Practice self-care: Prioritize self-care activities that promote emotional well-being. This can include activities like taking a bath, practicing relaxation techniques, engaging in hobbies, or spending time in nature.

Create a supportive environment: Surround yourself with a supportive community or join AIP-specific groups where you can share experiences, seek advice, and find encouragement from others who are on a similar journey.

Seek professional support: If emotional eating becomes a persistent challenge, consider seeking support from a therapist or counselor who can help you explore and address underlying emotional issues.

By implementing these strategies and focusing on self-care, mindfulness, and nourishing your body with nutrient-dense foods, you can effectively manage cravings and emotional eating during your AIP journey, promoting overall well-being and success. Remember that everyone's experience with the AIP is unique, so be patient with yourself and celebrate the progress you make along the way.

Foods to eliminate on the AIP diet:

Grains: Avoid all grains, including wheat, oats, rice, corn, and others.

Legumes: Exclude beans, lentils, soybeans, and peanuts.

Dairy: Remove all dairy products, including milk, cheese, yogurt, and butter.

Eggs: Eliminate eggs and foods containing eggs.

Nightshade vegetables: Avoid nightshade vegetables such as tomatoes, peppers, potatoes, and eggplants.

Nuts and seeds: Exclude all nuts and seeds, including almonds, walnuts, sesame seeds, and flaxseeds.

Refined sugars: Avoid all forms of refined sugar, including table sugar, high-fructose corn syrup, and artificial sweeteners.

Processed foods: Stay away from processed foods, including packaged snacks, chips, and pre-packaged meals.

Food additives: Avoid artificial additives, preservatives, and food colourings.

Foods to include on the AIP diet:

Vegetables: Focus on a wide variety of non-starchy vegetables, including leafy greens, broccoli, cauliflower, carrots, Brussels sprouts, and asparagus.

High-quality proteins: Consume grass-fed meat, wild-caught fish, and pasture-raised poultry. Include organ meats like liver and heart for added nutrient density.

Healthy fats: Use healthy fats like avocado, coconut oil, olive oil, and animal fats from pasture-raised sources.

Fruits: Enjoy fruits in moderation, focusing on low-sugar options such as berries, green apples, and pears.

Fermented foods: Include fermented foods like sauerkraut, kimchi, and coconut milk yogurt to support gut health.

Bone broth: Drink bone broth or use it as a base for soups and stews to provide collagen and gut-healing properties.

Herbs and spices: Use herbs and spices to add flavor and variety to your meals but be cautious of potential individual sensitivities.

Chapter 4: The Science Behind the AIP: Exploring the Link Between Inflammation, Diet, and Autoimmune Diseases

In this chapter, we will delve deeper into the scientific principles that underlie the Autoimmune Protocol (AIP). By examining the research and evidence supporting its efficacy in managing autoimmune conditions, we can gain a better understanding of the relationship between inflammation, diet, and autoimmune diseases.

The Scientific Rationale Behind the AIP:

The AIP is based on scientific research and theories that suggest a connection between diet, gut health, and autoimmune diseases. While the exact mechanisms are still being studied, several key principles support the scientific rationale behind the AIP:

Leaky gut theory: The AIP acknowledges the concept of "leaky gut," which suggests that increased intestinal permeability can lead to the passage of undigested food particles and toxins into the bloodstream. This can trigger an immune response and contribute to autoimmune conditions. By removing potential trigger foods and supporting gut healing, the AIP aims to reduce intestinal permeability and inflammation.

Inflammatory potential of certain foods: Foods, such as grains, legumes, dairy, and nightshade vegetables, contain compounds that may promote inflammation or trigger immune reactions in susceptible individuals. By eliminating these foods, the AIP aims to reduce the inflammatory load on the body and potentially alleviate symptoms.

Nutrient deficiencies and immune dysregulation: Autoimmune diseases are often associated with nutrient deficiencies and immune system dysregulation. The nutrient-dense foods emphasized in the AIP provide essential vitamins, minerals, and antioxidants that support immune function, reduce oxidative stress, and promote healing.

The Link Between Inflammation and Autoimmune Diseases:

Autoimmune diseases occur when the immune system mistakenly attacks healthy cells and tissues in the body. Inflammation, a natural immune response intended to protect against harmful stimuli, plays a significant role in the development and progression of autoimmune diseases.

Research has shown that chronic inflammation can contribute to the development of autoimmune conditions. Inflammation activates the immune system and can lead to the disruption of normal immune function, resulting in the immune system attacking healthy tissues. This sustained immune response perpetuates the cycle of inflammation and tissue damage, leading to the symptoms and progression of autoimmune diseases.

The Role of Diet in Autoimmune Diseases:

Emerging evidence suggests that diet can significantly impact the development and management of autoimmune diseases. The AIP focuses on removing potentially inflammatory foods and promoting nutrient-dense, anti-inflammatory options to support immune function and reduce inflammation.

16

Gluten and Dairy:

Gluten, a protein found in wheat and other grains, has been implicated in triggering autoimmune responses in susceptible individuals. Research suggests that gluten can increase intestinal permeability, allowing undigested proteins and other substances to enter the bloodstream and potentially activate the immune system.

In individuals with celiac disease, an autoimmune condition triggered by gluten, the immune system targets the small intestine, leading to inflammation and damage. However, even in individuals without celiac disease, gluten sensitivity may contribute to low-grade inflammation and exacerbate autoimmune symptoms.

Dairy products, particularly those containing lactose and casein, have also been associated with autoimmune diseases. Lactose intolerance, the inability to digest lactose, can lead to digestive symptoms and inflammation in susceptible individuals. Casein, a protein found in dairy, may stimulate immune responses and trigger inflammation in some people.

Furthermore, dairy products from conventionally raised cows may contain hormones and antibiotics that can disrupt gut health and promote inflammation. These factors make the exclusion of gluten and dairy essential in the AIP to minimize inflammation and support overall well-being.

Grains and Legumes:

The AIP eliminates grains and legumes due to their potential to contribute to inflammation and gut issues in individuals with autoimmune diseases. Grains such as wheat, corn, and rice contain lectins and phytic acid, which can irritate the gut lining and interfere with nutrient absorption.

Legumes, including beans, lentils, and soybeans, contain lectins and phytates that may also contribute to gut inflammation and impair digestion. Additionally, legumes are known to contain antinutrients that can hinder nutrient absorption and promote inflammation in susceptible individuals.

Nightshades:

Nightshade vegetables, such as tomatoes, potatoes, peppers, and eggplants, are excluded from the AIP due to their potential to exacerbate inflammation in some individuals. Nightshades contain alkaloids, including solanine and capsaicin, which may trigger immune responses and worsen symptoms in certain autoimmune conditions.

Although the impact of nightshades varies among individuals, eliminating them during the initial phase of the AIP can help identify potential triggers and allow for symptom improvement.

Eggs:

Eggs are temporarily eliminated on the AIP because they contain proteins that can be allergenic and potentially trigger immune responses in some individuals. The egg white, in particular, contains proteins such as albumin and ovomucoid, which are known to be common allergens. By removing eggs from the diet, individuals can identify whether eggs contribute to their symptoms and gradually reintroduce them later to assess their tolerance.

Nuts and Seeds:

Nuts and seeds, including almonds, walnuts, cashews, sesame seeds, and others, are excluded during the initial phase of the AIP. This is because they contain anti-nutrients like phytic acid and lectins, which can irritate the gut lining and interfere with nutrient absorption. Additionally, some individuals may be allergic or sensitive to specific nuts or seeds, and the elimination phase of the AIP helps identify these triggers. Over time, some people may reintroduce certain nuts and seeds based on their tolerance and individual needs.

Processed Foods, Sugar, and Additives:

Processed foods, high in refined sugars, unhealthy fats, and additives, are known to promote inflammation and contribute to various health issues. These foods often lack essential nutrients and contain artificial ingredients that can disrupt gut health and trigger immune responses.

Added sugars, including sucrose and high-fructose corn syrup, have been linked to increased inflammation, insulin resistance, and metabolic dysfunction. Artificial additives, such as artificial sweeteners, preservatives, and food colorings, can also provoke immune reactions and disrupt the gut microbiota, further exacerbating inflammation.

Excluding processed foods, sugar, and additives in the AIP helps reduce inflammation, stabilize blood sugar levels, and provide the body with nutrient-dense options necessary for healing and immune support.

Coffee and Chocolate:

Coffee and chocolate, although not inherently inflammatory, are temporarily eliminated on the AIP due to their potential to affect gut health and contribute to autoimmune symptoms. Coffee contains caffeine, which can stimulate the release of stress hormones and potentially disrupt the delicate balance of the immune system. Chocolate, particularly dark chocolate, contains compounds like theobromine, which may affect some individuals negatively. Eliminating coffee and chocolate during the initial phase of the AIP allows individuals to assess whether these items impact their symptoms.

Other Potential Trigger Foods:

While the AIP primarily focuses on the elimination of the aforementioned food groups, it's important to note that individual sensitivities can vary. Some people may find it beneficial to exclude additional foods that they suspect are triggering their symptoms. These may include high-lectin foods (such as legumes and certain grains), high-histamine foods (such as fermented foods and aged cheeses), and specific food additives or preservatives. The elimination and reintroduction process allows individuals to customize the AIP based on their specific needs and sensitivities.

Scientific research demonstrates the intricate relationship between inflammation, diet, and autoimmune diseases. The AIP addresses these connections by removing potentially inflammatory foods, promoting nutrient-dense options, and supporting gut health. By understanding the scientific principles underlying the AIP, individuals with autoimmune conditions can make informed dietary choices to manage their symptoms, reduce inflammation, and support their overall health and well-being. Through the exclusion of trigger foods and the inclusion of anti-inflammatory nutrients, the AIP aims to rebalance the immune system and provide a foundation for healing and managing autoimmune diseases.

Remember, the AIP elimination phase is not meant to be a permanent diet but rather a tool to identify trigger foods and alleviate symptoms. Once the initial phase is completed, foods are systematically reintroduced to determine an individual's tolerance and create a personalized long-term approach to managing autoimmune conditions. It's recommended to work with a healthcare professional or a registered dietitian experienced in autoimmune diseases to ensure nutritional adequacy and proper guidance throughout the process.

The Impact of Food on Autoimmune Diseases

The impact of food on autoimmune conditions is profound, as the health of the gut, particularly the gut microbiome and intestinal barrier, plays a critical role in the development and progression of autoimmune diseases. Emerging research suggests that diet plays a significant role in the development and management of autoimmune diseases. While genetics and other factors contribute to autoimmune conditions, certain dietary factors can influence immune function, inflammation levels, and gut health, all of which are interconnected with autoimmune diseases.

Mounting evidence suggests that specific foods can either trigger or exacerbate inflammation, contribute to gut dysbiosis (imbalance in gut bacteria), and compromise the integrity of the gut lining. These factors can potentially lead to an overactive immune response and the onset or progression of autoimmune conditions.

Gut Health and Its Connection to Autoimmune Diseases:

The health of the gut, specifically the gut microbiome and intestinal barrier, plays a crucial role in autoimmune diseases. The gut microbiome consists of trillions of microorganisms that interact with the immune system and influence various aspects of health.

When the gut microbiome is imbalanced or disrupted, a condition known as dysbiosis, it can trigger immune dysregulation and inflammation. Dysbiosis can be caused by factors such as poor diet, stress, infections, and antibiotic use. The compromised gut barrier, or leaky gut, allows the entry of harmful substances into the bloodstream, potentially leading to immune responses and autoimmune reactions.

Research suggests that interventions aimed at improving gut health, such as dietary modifications, probiotic supplementation, and lifestyle changes, can positively impact autoimmune diseases. By restoring a healthy gut microbiome and reducing gut permeability, it may be possible to modulate immune responses and alleviate symptoms associated with autoimmune conditions.

Understanding the impact of food on autoimmune diseases and recognizing the connection between diet, inflammation, and gut health is crucial for individuals seeking to manage their condition through dietary interventions. The Autoimmune Protocol (AIP) takes these factors into account by eliminating potential trigger foods and supporting gut healing to promote overall well-being and symptom relief.

Chapter 5: Getting Started with the AIP

Before embarking on the Autoimmune Protocol (AIP), it's important to make some preparations to set yourself up for success.

Assessing your readiness for the AIP:

Take the time to assess your commitment and readiness to follow the AIP. Understand the reasons why you want to try this protocol and how it aligns with your health goals. It may be helpful to consult with a healthcare professional or a registered dietitian who specialises in autoimmune conditions to get personalized guidance and support.

Setting realistic goals and expectations:

Set realistic goals for yourself and establish clear expectations. Understand that the AIP is a restrictive protocol that requires dedication and commitment. It may take time to see improvements, and individual results can vary. Being patient and having realistic expectations will help you stay motivated throughout the process.

Clearing your pantry and kitchen of non-compliant foods:

Go through your pantry, refrigerator, and kitchen to remove all non-compliant foods. Get rid of grains, legumes, dairy products, processed foods, refined sugars, industrial seed oils, nightshade vegetables, eggs, nuts and seeds, coffee, alcohol, and food additives. Stock up on AIP-friendly foods instead to ensure you have the necessary ingredients for your meals.

The Elimination Phase:

The first phase of the AIP is the elimination phase, where you remove all potentially problematic foods from your diet.

Identifying and eliminating AIP-restricted foods:

During the elimination phase, strictly avoid foods that are known to trigger inflammation and immune reactions. This includes grains, legumes, dairy, refined sugars, industrial seed oils, nightshade vegetables, eggs, nuts and seeds, coffee, alcohol, and food additives. Be diligent in reading food labels and be aware of hidden sources of these ingredients.

Sample meal plans and recipes for the elimination phase:

To help you get started, there are various resources available that provide sample meal plans and AIP-friendly recipes. These resources offer guidance on creating balanced meals that include quality meats, fish, vegetables (except nightshades), fruits, healthy fats, and fermented foods. Experiment with different flavors, herbs, and spices to keep your meals enjoyable and satisfying.

Building a Nutrient-Dense AIP Plate:

To ensure you're getting the necessary nutrients while following the Autoimmune Protocol (AIP), it's important to create balanced and nourishing meals.

Include quality protein: Prioritize grass-fed meats, wild-caught fish, and pastured poultry as sources of protein. These options provide essential amino acids and important micronutrients.

Load up on vegetables: Fill your plate with a variety of colorful non-starchy vegetables, such as leafy greens, cruciferous vegetables, root vegetables (except nightshades), and sea vegetables. These provide fiber, antioxidants, and a range of vitamins and minerals.

Include healthy fats: Incorporate healthy fats like avocado, coconut oil, olive oil, and animal fats. These fats support satiety, nutrient absorption, and provide essential fatty acids.

Don't forget about carbohydrates: While starchy vegetables are limited during the elimination phase, it's important to include carbohydrates from non-starchy vegetables and fruits to meet your energy needs.

Prioritize nutrient-dense foods: Choose foods that are rich in vitamins, minerals, and antioxidants. Include organ meats, bone broth, fermented foods, and sea vegetables to enhance nutrient intake.

While fruits are generally allowed on the AIP, they should be consumed in moderation, particularly for individuals with blood sugar regulation issues. It's important to choose low-glycemic fruits like berries and consume them as part of a balanced meal to minimize blood sugar spikes.

Fermented foods like sauerkraut, kimchi, and coconut milk yogurt are incredibly beneficial for gut health, as they provide probiotics that support a healthy balance of gut bacteria. Bone broth, rich in collagen and amino acids, is also strongly recommended for its gut-healing properties.

Key macronutrients and micronutrients to prioritize:

Macronutrients: Ensure you're getting an adequate amount of protein, healthy fats, and carbohydrates from compliant sources to support overall health and energy levels.

Micronutrients: Pay attention to nutrients like vitamin A, vitamin D, vitamin C, vitamin E, zinc, selenium, and omega-3 fatty acids. Include foods rich in these nutrients to support immune function, reduce inflammation, and promote healing.

Food sourcing and quality considerations:

Choose high-quality, organic, and locally sourced ingredients whenever possible. Opt for grass-fed and pasture-raised meats, wild-caught fish, and organic produce. Minimize exposure to pesticides, antibiotics, and hormones, which may contribute to inflammation and immune dysregulation.

Managing Cravings and Emotional Eating:

Additional tips for following the AIP diet:

- Read labels carefully: Avoid packaged foods that may contain hidden ingredients or additives not suitable for the AIP diet.
- Cook at home: Preparing meals at home using fresh, whole ingredients gives you control over what you eat and ensures compliance with the AIP guidelines.
- Plan and meal prep: Plan your meals in advance and batch cook to make it easier to stick to the diet during busy times.
- Stay hydrated: Drink plenty of water throughout the day to support overall health and hydration.
- Monitor your progress: Keep a food diary to track symptoms, including any reactions or improvements, as you reintroduce foods during the reintroduction phase.

- Seek professional guidance: Consider working with a healthcare professional or a nutritionist experienced in autoimmune conditions to receive personalised guidance and support.
- Familiarise yourself with the AIP guidelines and the list of allowed and restricted foods.
- Take inventory of your pantry and refrigerator, removing all non-compliant foods.
- Replace non-compliant foods with AIP-friendly alternatives like grass-fed meats, wild-caught fish, vegetables, and healthy fats.
- Create a weekly meal plan and corresponding shopping list to stay organized and ensure you have necessary ingredients.
- Consider gradually transitioning to the AIP by eliminating non-compliant foods in stages.
- Seek support from online communities or support groups where you can share experiences and receive guidance.
- Stay committed and focused on your goals, celebrating small milestones along the way.
- Listen to your body and make adjustments as needed to suit your individual needs.

- Work with a healthcare professional or registered dietitian experienced in autoimmune conditions for personalised support and guidance.

Chapter 6: Food Preparation for Success

Food preparation plays a crucial role in the successful implementation of the Autoimmune Protocol (AIP). By prepping your meals ahead of time, you can experience several benefits. Firstly, it saves you time, as having pre-prepared meals and ingredients reduces the time spent in the kitchen, especially on busy days. Secondly, it ensures compliance with the AIP guidelines. When you prepare meals in advance, you have control over the ingredients, ensuring that all your meals are AIP-friendly. This helps you stay on track and supports your health goals. Additionally, food preparation reduces decision fatigue. When your meals are pre-planned and prepped, you eliminate the need to make food-related decisions on the spot. This reduces stress and minimizes the chances of deviating from the AIP. Lastly, food preparation promotes consistency, which is crucial for achieving desired health outcomes. Even on hectic days or when cravings strike, having pre-prepared meals helps you stay on track with the AIP.

Practical Tips for Food Prep

To streamline your food preparation process, consider the following tips:

Plan your meals: Create a weekly meal plan outlining breakfast, lunch, dinner, and snacks. This helps you stay organized and ensures that you have a variety of nutrient-dense AIP meals throughout the week.

Batch cook: Dedicate a specific time during the week to batch cook staple ingredients like proteins, vegetables, and AIP-approved sauces. This allows you to assemble meals quickly during the week.

Use meal prep containers: Invest in quality, food-safe containers to store prepped ingredients and meals. Divided containers can be particularly useful for storing different components of a meal.

Wash and chop vegetables: Wash and chop vegetables in advance to save time. Store them in airtight containers or bags to maintain freshness.

Portion and freeze: If you have limited time during the week, consider portioning out and freezing pre-cooked meals or ingredients. This way, you can simply thaw and reheat when needed.

Prep snacks: Prepare AIP-friendly snacks, such as homemade energy balls, chopped fruit, or vegetable sticks with dip, in advance. This ensures that you have convenient and healthy snack options readily available.

Utilize kitchen appliances: Use tools like slow cookers, pressure cookers, or Instant Pots to save time and effortlessly prepare meals.

Chop and prep ingredients in advance: Wash, chop, and store vegetables and fruits for easy access during the week. Pre-portion snacks and meals for grab-and-go convenience.

Batch cooking tips:

- Cook large batches of proteins like chicken, beef, or fish that can be used in various meals throughout the week.
- Roast a sheet pan of mixed vegetables, such as carrots, Brussels sprouts, and sweet potatoes.
- Prepare big batches of soups, stews, or casseroles that can be portioned and frozen for later use.
- Make AIP-friendly sauces, dressings, or marinades in larger quantities and store them in the refrigerator for quick flavor additions to meals.

Storing and freezing AIP-friendly meals for convenience:

Invest in airtight containers or freezer-friendly bags to store pre-portioned meals. Label and date your containers for easy identification. Freeze meals that you won't consume within a few days to maintain freshness. Thaw frozen meals in the refrigerator overnight.

Food preparation is a fundamental aspect of successfully following the AIP. By investing time in meal preparation, you can save time, ensure compliance with the AIP, reduce decision fatigue, and promote consistency in your dietary choices. Plan your meals, batch cook, use meal prep containers, wash and chop vegetables, portion and freeze meals, and prepare snacks in advance. By following these practical tips, you'll be well-prepared to nourish your body with delicious and compliant AIP meals throughout the week. Remember, food preparation is an investment in your health and a valuable tool for maintaining success on the AIP journey.

Chapter 8: Managing Social Situations on the AIP

When following the Autoimmune Protocol (AIP), social situations can pose unique challenges. Navigating gatherings, dining out, and other social events while adhering to the AIP may require some additional planning and communication. In this chapter, we will explore practical strategies and tips to help you feel confident and empowered in social settings while maintaining the integrity of the AIP. By proactively managing social situations, you can enjoy meaningful connections and stay on track with your health goals.

Communicating Your Dietary Needs:

One of the keys to successfully managing social situations on the AIP is effectively communicating your dietary needs to others. Inform your friends, family, and hosts about your dietary restrictions in advance, explaining the reasons behind your choices. Share resources or information about the AIP to help them understand your situation better. By communicating openly and honestly, you can set realistic expectations and encourage support from those around you.

Offering to Contribute:

When attending social gatherings or potluck events, offer to bring an AIP-friendly dish or two. This ensures that you will have at least one dish you can enjoy while also introducing others to delicious and healthy AIP-compliant options. Choose recipes that are flavorful, visually appealing, and resemble familiar dishes to make them more accessible and appealing to everyone.

Planning Ahead:

If you're attending an event where you don't have control over the food served, plan ahead by eating a satisfying AIP-compliant meal before you go. This will help you feel less tempted by non-compliant foods and ensure that you're not overly hungry when faced with limited options. Additionally, consider carrying portable AIP-friendly snacks or a small meal with you, such as a protein bar, cut vegetables, or a homemade AIP snack, to have a backup option in case there are no suitable choices available.

Communicating with Restaurants:

Dining out can be challenging on the AIP, but with proper communication, it can still be an enjoyable experience. Call ahead to the restaurant and inquire about their flexibility in accommodating dietary restrictions. Explain your needs and ask if they can modify dishes or offer alternatives. Many restaurants are becoming more aware of dietary restrictions and may be willing to accommodate your needs. If necessary, ask for simple modifications like steamed vegetables, grilled protein, or a salad with dressing on the side.

Focus on the Social Connection:

While food is often a central aspect of social events, remember that the primary purpose is to connect with others. Shift your focus from the food to the conversations, laughter, and enjoyment of the company. By emphasizing the social aspect, you can reduce the feeling of deprivation and better appreciate the meaningful interactions.

Seek Support from Loved Ones:

Share your AIP journey with loved ones and ask for their support. Having friends and family who understand your health goals and are willing to accommodate your dietary needs can make social situations more comfortable. Engage in open conversations, educate them about the AIP, and express your gratitude for their understanding. Their support will help you feel more at ease and less isolated in social settings.

Practicing Mindful Eating:

When you're at social events, practice mindful eating by paying attention to your body's hunger and fullness cues. Take your time to savor each bite, focusing on the flavors and textures of the AIP-compliant foods you are enjoying. This mindful approach can help you feel more satisfied and prevent overeating or feeling deprived.

Developing Coping Strategies:

In social situations, you may encounter moments of temptation or frustration. Develop coping strategies to manage these challenges effectively. Engage in deep breathing exercises, visualize your health goals, or repeat positive affirmations to stay focused and motivated. Having a repertoire of strategies will empower you to overcome obstacles and maintain your commitment to the AIP.

Finding Supportive Communities:

Connect with online AIP communities, support groups, or forums where you can interact with others on a similar journey. These communities provide a space to share experiences, seek advice, and find encouragement. Engaging with like-minded individuals who understand the challenges of the AIP can provide a sense of belonging and support during social situations.

Managing social situations on the AIP requires proactive planning, effective communication, and a positive mindset. By openly communicating your dietary needs, offering to contribute AIP-friendly dishes, planning ahead, and focusing on the social connection, you can navigate social events with confidence and maintain your commitment to the AIP. Remember, with preparation, support, and mindfulness, you can enjoy meaningful social interactions while staying true to your health goals.

Chapter 9: The Reintroduction Process: Individualizing the Autoimmune Protocol (AIP) for Long-Term Success

In this chapter, we will explore the critical phase of the Autoimmune Protocol (AIP) known as the reintroduction process. While the elimination phase of the AIP helps individuals identify trigger foods and reduce inflammation, the reintroduction phase allows for the customisation of the diet based on individual tolerances and preferences. Understanding the reintroduction process, including the recommended timeline, waiting periods, portion sizes, and tips, is essential for long-term success with the AIP.

The Purpose of Reintroduction:

The reintroduction phase of the AIP serves two primary purposes: to identify trigger foods and to expand the diet to enhance variety and nutrient intake. By systematically reintroducing eliminated foods, individuals can determine which specific foods may be causing adverse reactions or symptoms. This knowledge empowers individuals to create a personalised, sustainable diet that accommodates their unique sensitivities and preferences while still supporting their autoimmune health.

The Reintroduction Timeline:

The duration of the elimination phase of the AIP can vary depending on individual circumstances and needs. However, a commonly recommended timeframe for the elimination phase is typically around 30 to 60 days. This period allows for the reduction of inflammation, gut healing, and symptom improvement.

Once the elimination phase is complete, the reintroduction phase begins. It's essential to approach reintroduction systematically and gradually to accurately assess individual responses to each reintroduced food. Here is a general timeline for the reintroduction process:

Start with the Basics:

Begin by reintroducing the most basic and well-tolerated foods first. These include non-triggering foods such as white rice, which is gluten-free and easily digestible. Consume a small portion, such as half a cup, and observe for any immediate or delayed reactions over the next 24 to 48 hours. Keep a detailed food journal to track any symptoms or changes.

Introduce One Food Group at a Time:

After establishing a baseline with the basic foods, reintroduce one food group at a time. For example, you can start with eggs, nuts and seeds, nightshades, or dairy. Choose one food from the group and consume a small amount, such as a quarter of a serving. Preferably, consume the food in its purest form, without any added ingredients. Observe for any adverse reactions over the next three days.

Waiting Periods:

When reintroducing foods on the Autoimmune Protocol (AIP), it is generally recommended to wait at least three to seven days between introducing each new food. This waiting period allows you to observe and monitor your body's response to the reintroduced food. I personally would wait seven days to provide sufficient time to evaluate any potential reactions or symptoms that may arise after reintroducing a specific food. This waiting period helps ensure that you have enough time to assess the impact of the food on your body before moving on to the next reintroduction.

Assess Individual Tolerance:

During this waiting period, it's important to pay attention to any changes in your symptoms, such as digestive issues, skin reactions, joint pain, fatigue, or changes in mood. Keeping a food diary can be helpful in tracking and documenting any symptoms or reactions that occur during the reintroduction process.

If you experience a reaction or symptoms after reintroducing a food, it's recommended to wait until the symptoms subside before moving on to the next reintroduction. This allows your body time to recover and provides a clear baseline for evaluating the effects of the next food reintroduction.

Portion Sizes:

When reintroducing foods, start with small portions to assess individual tolerance. Gradually increase the portion sizes over time, as long as no adverse reactions occur. Pay attention to portion sizes that elicit symptoms, as this can indicate a specific threshold of tolerance for that particular food.

Customise the Diet:

Based on the individual's responses during reintroduction, the diet can be customized to include tolerated foods while avoiding trigger foods. Some individuals may find that they can reintroduce certain foods without any adverse effects, while others may need to continue avoiding specific foods that consistently trigger symptoms. This customization ensures that the diet remains personalized and supportive of individual health goals.

Chapter 10: The Healing Power of Fasting and Intermittent Fasting

Fasting has been shown to have a profound influence on inflammation within the body. When you fast, the body undergoes several physiological changes that impact the immune system and inflammation levels. One of these changes is the reduction in pro-inflammatory markers, which can help alleviate symptoms associated with autoimmune conditions.

The correlation between fasting and gut health is an intriguing area of study that is gaining attention among researchers and health professionals. Fasting can have several positive effects on gut health, including promoting gut microbiome balance, reducing inflammation in the gut, and supporting intestinal barrier function.

Gut Microbiome Balance:

The gut microbiome refers to the trillions of microorganisms residing in the digestive tract, including beneficial bacteria, viruses, and fungi. A healthy gut microbiome is crucial for proper digestion, nutrient absorption, immune function, and overall well-being. Imbalances in the gut microbiome have been linked to various health conditions, including autoimmune diseases and gastrointestinal disorders.

Fasting has been shown to have a positive impact on the gut microbiome. Animal studies have demonstrated that fasting can lead to shifts in the gut microbial composition, favoring the growth of beneficial bacteria. These changes can improve gut health, enhance the diversity of the microbiome, and support a balanced ecosystem in the gut.

Reduced Gut Inflammation:

Inflammation in the gut, often referred to as gut inflammation, is a common feature of many gastrointestinal disorders, including inflammatory bowel disease (IBD) and leaky gut syndrome. Chronic inflammation in the gut can damage the intestinal lining, disrupt gut barrier function, and contribute to the development or exacerbation of autoimmune conditions.

Fasting has been shown to reduce gut inflammation by modulating the immune response and suppressing pro-inflammatory cytokines. By reducing inflammation in the gut, fasting may alleviate symptoms associated with gastrointestinal disorders and promote overall gut health.

Intestinal Barrier Function:

The intestinal barrier serves as a protective barrier between the inside of the gut and the rest of the body. It plays a crucial role in preventing harmful substances, toxins, and undigested food particles from entering the bloodstream. When the intestinal barrier becomes compromised, as in the case of leaky gut syndrome, it can lead to increased inflammation and immune dysregulation.

Fasting has been found to support intestinal barrier function by enhancing the production of tight junction proteins, which help maintain the integrity of the gut lining. This reinforcement of the intestinal barrier can reduce the permeability of the gut and prevent the passage of harmful substances into the bloodstream, thereby promoting gut health.

Autophagy: Cellular Cleansing and Repair:

During a fast, a process called autophagy is triggered within the body. Autophagy is a natural cellular mechanism where damaged or dysfunctional cells are broken down and recycled. By enhancing autophagy through fasting, the body can remove malfunctioning immune cells and reduce overall inflammation. This process supports cellular cleansing and repair, contributing to the healing of autoimmune conditions.

In simple terms, it can be thought of as a cellular cleaning and recycling system.

Modulating the Immune System:

Intermittent fasting has shown promising effects on immune system regulation. It helps balance the activity of immune cells, reducing the production of pro-inflammatory cytokines and promoting the production of anti-inflammatory molecules. By modulating the immune response, IF may alleviate symptoms associated with autoimmune conditions and create a more balanced immune environment.

Modulating the immune system through fasting refers to the ability of fasting to influence and regulate immune responses in the body. Fasting has been found to have immune-modulating effects, promoting a balanced and efficient immune system. Let's delve into the details:

Immune System Balance:

Fasting can help restore balance to the immune system. It has been observed that fasting can reduce excessive immune activity, such as inflammation, by suppressing pro-inflammatory pathways. This downregulation of immune responses during fasting can be beneficial for individuals with autoimmune conditions or chronic inflammatory diseases.

During fasting, the body taps into its energy reserves and breaks down older or damaged cells for energy. This includes immune cells, particularly older or dysfunctional ones. As a result, fasting promotes the regeneration of new immune cells from stem cells, potentially rejuvenating the immune system.

Fasting has been shown to enhance the resilience of the immune system. It can promote the production of antioxidants and increase the activity of enzymes that protect cells from oxidative stress. This improved antioxidant capacity and cellular protection can enhance the immune system's ability to defend against infections and diseases.

The Role of Intermittent Fasting:

Intermittent fasting (IF) is an eating pattern that alternates between periods of fasting and eating. Unlike prolonged fasting, IF offers a more manageable and sustainable approach. By restricting the eating window, IF allows the body to experience the benefits of fasting while still providing essential nutrients during the feeding period.

Getting Started with Intermittent Fasting:

- Choose an IF protocol: Select an intermittent fasting protocol that aligns with your lifestyle and preferences. Popular options include the 16/8 method (fasting for 16 hours and eating within an 8-hour window) or the 5:2 method (eating normally for five days and restricting calorie intake on two non-consecutive days).

- Gradual adjustment: Ease into intermittent fasting by gradually extending the fasting period. Start with a shorter fasting window and gradually increase it over time to allow your body to adapt.

- Stay hydrated: Drink plenty of water during fasting periods to stay hydrated and support the body's detoxification processes.

- Nutrient-dense meals: When you break your fast, focus on consuming balanced, nutrient-dense meals that include a variety of vegetables, lean proteins, healthy fats, and complex carbohydrates.

- Listen to your body: Pay attention to how your body responds to fasting. If you experience any adverse effects or discomfort, adjust your fasting schedule or seek guidance from a healthcare professional.

In addition to the potential benefits of fasting and intermittent fasting for inflammation and autoimmune conditions, these practices can also be helpful for individuals following the Autoimmune Protocol (AIP) diet. The AIP diet restricts many common breakfast options, making it challenging to find suitable and satisfying morning meals.

If you find the breakfast options limited with the AIP diet, it might be worth considering intermittent fasting and skipping breakfast altogether. By extending the fasting period in the morning, you can simplify your meal planning and focus on creating nutrient-dense and compliant meals during your eating window. This approach allows you to maximize the benefits of fasting while still adhering to the dietary restrictions of the AIP protocol.

By combining the principles of intermittent fasting and the AIP diet, you can optimize your healing journey and potentially experience improvements in symptoms, inflammation levels, and overall well-being. As always, it is crucial to prioritize your health and make decisions that best support your unique needs and circumstances.

Chapter 11: Stress Management and Sleep:

Stress and lack of quality sleep can have a significant impact on autoimmune conditions. Implementing strategies to manage stress and improve sleep can support your overall well-being and enhance the effectiveness of the Autoimmune Protocol (AIP).

The impact of stress and lack of sleep on autoimmune conditions:

Stress can trigger immune system dysregulation and inflammation, exacerbating autoimmune symptoms. Additionally, inadequate sleep can impair immune function, increase inflammation, and disrupt hormonal balance, further compromising the body's ability to heal.

Techniques for stress reduction and relaxation:

Mindfulness meditation: Practice mindfulness meditation to cultivate present-moment awareness and reduce stress. Apps or guided meditation resources can assist you in establishing a regular practice.

Deep breathing exercises: Engage in deep breathing exercises to activate the body's relaxation response. Breathing deeply into your diaphragm and exhaling fully can help calm the nervous system.

Gentle movement practices: Explore gentle movement practices such as yoga, tai chi, or qigong. These activities promote relaxation, improve flexibility, and reduce stress.

Stress-reducing activities: Engage in activities that you find enjoyable and relaxing, such as taking walks in nature, listening to music, reading, or engaging in hobbies.

Promoting quality sleep for optimal healing:

Establish a bedtime routine: Create a consistent bedtime routine that includes activities that signal to your body that it's time to wind down. This may include reading a book, taking a warm bath, or practicing relaxation techniques.

Create a sleep-friendly environment: Ensure your sleep environment is conducive to quality sleep. Keep the room cool, dark, and quiet. Consider using earplugs, an eye mask, or white noise machines if needed.

Limit electronic device usage before bed: The blue light emitted by electronic devices can disrupt sleep. Avoid using electronic devices, such as smartphones or tablets, for at least an hour before bed.

Stick to a consistent sleep schedule: Establish regular bed and wake times to regulate your body's internal clock. Consistency in sleep patterns can improve sleep quality.

Physical Activity and Movement:

Regular exercise and movement can have numerous benefits for autoimmune health. It's important to choose activities that align with your energy levels and abilities, and find ways to incorporate movement into your daily routine.

The benefits of exercise for autoimmune health:

Boosted immune function: Regular exercise can enhance immune function, reduce inflammation, and support overall immune system health.

45

Improved mood and mental well-being: Exercise releases endorphins, which can improve mood and reduce symptoms of anxiety and depression.

Increased energy and stamina: Engaging in regular physical activity can improve energy levels and reduce fatigue.

Enhanced cardiovascular health: Exercise can strengthen the heart and improve cardiovascular health, reducing the risk of associated conditions.

Choosing suitable activities for your energy levels and abilities:

Listen to your body: Pay attention to your energy levels and any physical limitations. Choose activities that are appropriate for your current abilities and gradually increase intensity or duration as you feel comfortable.

Seek professional guidance: Consult with a healthcare professional or a qualified exercise specialist who can provide guidance on suitable exercises and modifications tailored to your condition.

Consider low-impact activities: If you have joint pain or limited mobility, low-impact activities like swimming, cycling, or gentle yoga may be more suitable and less likely to exacerbate symptoms.

Incorporating movement into your daily routine:

Find opportunities for movement: Look for ways to incorporate movement into your daily routine. Take short walks during breaks, use stairs instead of elevators, or engage in household chores or gardening.

Break up sedentary time: If you have a sedentary job, make an effort to take regular movement breaks. Stand up, stretch, or do simple exercises to avoid prolonged sitting.

Seeking Support and Accountability:

Building a support network and seeking professional guidance can be invaluable during your AIP journey. Support and accountability can help you stay motivated, navigate challenges, and celebrate your progress.

Building a support network of friends, family, or online communities:

Share your journey: Openly communicate with your friends and family about your AIP journey, explaining the reasons behind your dietary and lifestyle choices. Seek their understanding and support.

Join online communities: Participate in online forums, social media groups, or AIP-specific communities where you can connect with others who are following a similar path. Share experiences, ask questions, and find encouragement from like-minded individuals.

Set realistic goals: Break down your long-term goals into smaller, achievable milestones. Celebrate each milestone reached to stay motivated and encouraged.

Track your progress: Keep a journal or use tracking apps to monitor your symptoms, food intake, exercise, and overall well-being. Seeing improvements over time can inspire you to continue on your AIP journey.

Reward yourself: Treat yourself to non-food rewards when you achieve your goals or make progress. This could be anything from buying a new book, enjoying a spa day, or engaging in a favorite hobby.

Chapter 12: Example of a Weekly Meal Planner and Shopping List:

Here's an example of a weekly meal planner and shopping list to give you an idea of how to structure your AIP meals:

Weekly Meal Plan:

Day 1:

Breakfast: Sweet potato hash with ground turkey, kale, and herbs.

Lunch: Mixed greens salad with grilled salmon, sliced cucumber, and olive oil dressing.

Dinner: Baked chicken thighs with roasted carrots and steamed broccoli.

Day 2:

Breakfast: AIP-friendly smoothie made with coconut milk, spinach, blueberries, and collagen peptides.

Lunch: Cabbage and ground beef skillet with onion, garlic, and turmeric.

Dinner: Baked cod with roasted asparagus and mashed cauliflower.

Day 3:

Breakfast: Sweet potato hash with ground turkey, kale, and herbs.

Lunch: Butternut squash soup topped with cooked shrimp.

Dinner: Grass-fed beef burger wrapped in lettuce leaves, served with baked sweet potato fries.

Day 4:

Breakfast: Zucchini and carrot fritters with avocado slices.

Lunch: Mixed greens salad with grilled chicken, sliced beets, and lemon-tahini dressing.

Dinner: Oven-roasted turkey breast with sautéed Brussels sprouts and baked plantains.

Day 5:

Breakfast: AIP-friendly breakfast bowl with sliced avocado, cooked bacon, and arugula.

Lunch: Coconut milk-based chicken curry with cauliflower rice.

Dinner: Baked salmon with roasted butternut squash and steamed kale.

Day 6:

Breakfast: AIP-friendly breakfast bowl with sliced avocado, cooked bacon, and arugula.

Lunch: Tuna salad with mixed greens, cucumber, and olive oil dressing.

Dinner: Lemon herb roasted chicken with roasted broccoli and mashed turnips.

Day 7:

Breakfast: AIP-friendly smoothie made with coconut milk, kale, mango, and collagen peptides.

Lunch: Turkey lettuce wraps filled with avocado, shredded carrots, and sliced radishes.

Dinner: Baked halibut with sautéed zucchini noodles and garlic.

Shopping List:

Chicken (thighs, breast)

Salmon

Cod

Shrimp

Ground beef

Ground turkey

Grass-fed beef burger patties

Turkey breast

Bacon

Tuna

Coconut milk

Avocado

Sweet potatoes

Butternut squash

Zucchini

Carrots

Spinach

Kale

Mixed greens

Cabbage

Brussels sprouts

Asparagus

Broccoli

Cauliflower

Radishes

Beets

Lemon

Fresh herbs (such as parsley, cilantro, basil)

Coconut oil

Olive oil

Salt

Turmeric

Garlic

Collagen peptides (optional)

Blueberries

Mango

Chapter 13: Recipes

AIP Vegetable Fritters:

Ingredients:

2 cups grated zucchini

1 cup grated carrot

1/4 cup finely chopped onion

1/4 cup coconut flour

2 tablespoons coconut oil (melted)

1/2 teaspoon garlic powder

1/2 teaspoon dried herbs (such as thyme or parsley)

Salt to taste

Cooking fat (such as coconut oil or avocado oil) for frying

Instructions:

In a large bowl, combine grated zucchini, grated carrot, chopped onion, coconut flour, melted coconut oil, garlic powder, dried herbs, and salt. Mix well until the ingredients are evenly combined.

Allow the mixture to sit for 5 minutes to allow the coconut flour to absorb some moisture.

Heat a skillet over medium heat and add enough cooking fat to coat the bottom of the pan.

Take a spoonful of the fritter mixture and place it in the skillet, then flatten it with the back of the spoon to form a fritter shape. Repeat with the remaining mixture, leaving some space between each fritter.

Cook the fritters for about 3-4 minutes on each side or until they turn golden brown and crispy.

Once cooked, transfer the fritters to a plate lined with a paper towel to absorb any excess oil.

Serve the vegetable fritters warm. You can enjoy them as is or pair them with some AIP-friendly sauce or dip.

Sweet Potato Hash:

Ingredients:

2 medium sweet potatoes, peeled and grated

1/2 cup finely chopped onion

2 cloves garlic, minced

2 tablespoons cooking fat (such as coconut oil or avocado oil)

1 teaspoon dried thyme

1/2 teaspoon sea salt

1/4 teaspoon black pepper (omit for strict AIP)

Instructions:

Heat the cooking fat in a large skillet over medium heat.

Add the chopped onion and minced garlic to the skillet and sauté until they become fragrant and slightly softened, about 2-3 minutes.

Add the grated sweet potatoes, dried thyme, sea salt, and black pepper (if using) to the skillet. Mix well to combine all the ingredients.

Cook the sweet potato hash, stirring occasionally, for about 10-12 minutes or until the sweet potatoes are cooked through and slightly crispy.

Once the sweet potato hash is cooked to your desired texture, remove it from the heat.

Serve the sweet potato hash as a side dish or as a base for other ingredients. It pairs well with cooked protein sources like chicken, beef, or fish.

Feel free to modify the recipe by adding other AIP-friendly vegetables or herbs that you enjoy. The cooking time may vary depending on the thickness of the sweet potato shreds and desired texture.

AIP Chicken Nuggets with Sweet Potato (Using Ground Chicken or Turkey):

Ingredients:

1 pound ground chicken or ground turkey

1/2 cup coconut flour

1 teaspoon garlic powder

1 teaspoon onion powder

1/2 teaspoon dried oregano

1/2 teaspoon dried thyme

1/2 teaspoon sea salt

1/2 cup cooked and mashed sweet potato

1/4 cup coconut oil, for frying

Instructions:

In a mixing bowl, combine the ground chicken or ground turkey, coconut flour, garlic powder, onion powder, dried oregano, dried thyme, and sea salt. Mix well until all the ingredients are evenly incorporated.

Add the mashed sweet potato to the bowl and continue mixing until the sweet potato is well distributed throughout the mixture.

Take a portion of the mixture and shape it into a nugget form, about 1-2 inches in size. Repeat with the remaining mixture.

Heat the coconut oil in a large skillet over medium heat.

Place the shaped chicken or turkey nuggets into the skillet, leaving some space between each piece. Cook in batches if necessary.

Cook the nuggets for about 5-6 minutes on each side, or until they are cooked through and golden brown.

Once cooked, transfer the chicken or turkey nuggets to a plate lined with a paper towel to absorb any excess oil.

Serve the AIP chicken or turkey nuggets with sweet potato warm as a main dish or as a fun finger food. Pair them with an AIP-friendly dipping sauce such as guacamole or homemade mayonnaise.

AIP Cauliflower Fried Rice:

Ingredients:

1 small head cauliflower, riced

1 tablespoon coconut oil

2 cloves garlic, minced

1 cup diced carrots

1 cup diced zucchini

1 cup chopped broccoli

2 green onions, thinly sliced

2 tablespoons coconut aminos

Sea salt to taste

Instructions:

Heat coconut oil in a large skillet or wok over medium heat.

Add the garlic and cook until fragrant.

Add the carrots, zucchini, and broccoli, and cook until slightly tender.

Add the riced cauliflower and cook until it is heated through.

Stir in the green onions and coconut aminos.

Season with sea salt to taste.

Remove from heat and serve as a nutritious side dish or add cooked protein of your choice for a complete meal.

AIP Baked Chicken with Herbs:

Ingredients:

4 bone-in, skin-on chicken thighs

2 tablespoons extra-virgin olive oil

1 teaspoon dried thyme

1 teaspoon dried rosemary

1 teaspoon dried sage

Sea salt to taste

Instructions:

Preheat the oven to 400°F (200°C).

Place the chicken thighs on a baking sheet lined with parchment paper.

Drizzle the chicken thighs with olive oil and rub to coat them evenly.

In a small bowl, mix together the dried thyme, dried rosemary, dried sage, and sea salt.

Sprinkle the herb mixture over the chicken thighs, pressing gently to adhere.

Bake for about 35-40 minutes, or until the chicken is cooked through and the skin is crispy.

Serve the baked chicken thighs with a side of roasted vegetables or a salad.

AIP Turmeric Ginger Carrot Soup:

Ingredients:

1 tablespoon coconut oil

1 onion, chopped

3 cloves garlic, minced

1-inch piece of fresh ginger, grated

4 cups chopped carrots

4 cups bone broth or vegetable broth

1 teaspoon ground turmeric

Sea salt to taste

Instructions:

Heat coconut oil in a large pot over medium heat.

Add the onion, garlic, and grated ginger, and sauté until fragrant.

Add the chopped carrots and cook for a few minutes.

Pour in the bone broth or vegetable broth, and bring to a boil.

Reduce the heat and simmer until the carrots are tender.

Using an immersion blender or countertop blender, puree the soup until smooth.

Stir in the ground turmeric, and season with sea salt to taste.

Serve the turmeric ginger carrot soup warm, garnished with fresh herbs if desired.

AIP Sheet Pan Chicken and Vegetables:

Ingredients:

4 boneless, skinless chicken breasts

2 cups chopped sweet potatoes

2 cups Brussels sprouts, halved

1 cup sliced carrots

2 tablespoons extra-virgin olive oil

1 teaspoon dried thyme

1 teaspoon dried rosemary

Sea salt to taste

Instructions:

Preheat the oven to 400°F (200°C).

Place the chicken breasts, sweet potatoes, Brussels sprouts, and carrots on a baking sheet.

Drizzle with olive oil and sprinkle with dried thyme, dried rosemary, and sea salt.

Toss everything together to coat evenly.

Bake for about 25-30 minutes, or until the chicken is cooked through and the vegetables are tender.

Serve the sheet pan chicken and vegetables hot as a complete meal.

AIP Salmon with Roasted Root Vegetables:

Ingredients:

2 salmon fillets

2 cups chopped beets

2 cups chopped turnips

2 cups chopped parsnips

2 tablespoons extra-virgin olive oil

1 teaspoon dried dill

Sea salt to taste

Instructions:

Preheat the oven to 400°F (200°C).

Place the salmon fillets and chopped root vegetables on a baking sheet.

Drizzle with olive oil and sprinkle with dried dill and sea salt.

Toss everything together to coat evenly.

Bake for about 20-25 minutes, or until the salmon is cooked to your desired doneness and the vegetables are tender.

Serve the salmon with roasted root vegetables and enjoy.

AIP Beef Stir-Fry with Cauliflower Rice:

Ingredients:

1 pound grass-fed ground beef

1 head cauliflower, riced

2 cups sliced mushrooms

1 cup chopped bok choy

1 cup sliced bell peppers

2 tablespoons coconut aminos

1 tablespoon grated ginger

2 cloves garlic, minced

2 tablespoons coconut oil

Sea salt to taste

Instructions:

Heat coconut oil in a large skillet or wok over medium heat.

Add the ground beef and cook until browned.

Add the mushrooms, bok choy, bell peppers, grated ginger, and minced garlic. Sauté until the vegetables are tender.

Stir in the coconut aminos and season with sea salt to taste.

In a separate skillet, heat coconut oil over medium heat and sauté the cauliflower rice until tender.

Serve the beef stir-fry over the cauliflower rice and enjoy.

AIP Banana Pancakes:

Ingredients:

2 ripe bananas

4 tablespoons coconut flour

4 tablespoons arrowroot flour

4 tablespoons coconut milk

2 teaspoons lemon juice

1/2 teaspoon baking soda

Pinch of sea salt

Coconut oil (for cooking)

Instructions:

In a mixing bowl, mash the ripe bananas until smooth.

Add the coconut flour, arrowroot flour, coconut milk, lemon juice, baking soda, and sea salt to the bowl. Mix well until a batter forms.

Heat a non-stick skillet or griddle over medium heat and add a small amount of coconut oil to coat the surface.

Spoon about 1/4 cup of the pancake batter onto the skillet for each pancake.

Cook the pancakes for about 2-3 minutes on each side, or until golden brown.

Repeat with the remaining batter, adding more coconut oil to the skillet as needed.

Serve the AIP banana pancakes warm with your choice of AIP-friendly toppings such as fresh berries, coconut cream, or drizzled honey (if tolerated).

www.ingramcontent.com/pod-product-compliance
Lightning Source LLC
Chambersburg PA
CBHW072257310526
45795CB00012B/1707